HELP FOR
BED WETTING

95

HELP FOR
BED WETTING

ROY MEADOW, MA, BM, FRCP, DObstRCOG, DCH
Professor of Paediatrics and Child Health and Honorary Consultant
Paediatrician, St James's University Hospital, Leeds

CHURCHILL LIVINGSTONE
EDINBURGH LONDON MELBOURNE AND NEW YORK 1980

CHURCHILL LIVINGSTONE
Medical Division of Longman Group Limited

Distributed in the United States of America by Churchill
Livingstone Inc., 19 West 44th Street, New York, N.Y. 10036,
and by associated companies, branches and representatives
throughout the world.

First published 1980

ISBN 0 443 02236 4

British Library Cataloguing in Publication Data
Meadow, Samuel Roy
  Help for bed wetting
  1. Enuresis
  I. Title
  616.6'3   RC 564   80-40329

Printed in Singapore
by Singapore Offset Printing Pte Ltd

ACKNOWLEDGEMENTS

The figures were prepared by Mr Brian Emmison and the Medical Illustration Department at St James's University Hospital, Leeds. I am grateful to my assistant Mrs Wendy Pearson.

CONTENTS

Bed wetting

It is common

It causes much unhappiness

But there are ways of stopping it

BED WETTING CAN BE CURED

HOW COMMON IS IT?

At the age of 5 years 15 per cent of children, or about one in seven, wet the bed. Many of them wet the bed nearly every night. Most have not had a dry period longer than a day or two. By the age of 10 years 7 per cent, or one in fourteen, wet the bed. By the age of 15 only about 1 per cent of children wet the bed.

So, it is very common in young school children, and less common in teenagers (but nevertheless one can estimate that there are more than five thousand 15-year-olds in the United Kingdom who are troubled with bed wetting).

Bed wetting occurs in both sexes, though in school children it is twice as common in boys as girls.

The good news is that bed wetting tends to disappear with time. Even without any special treatment one in seven of school children who wet the bed will become dry during the next year. For teenagers the proportion becoming dry is greater. With special help the proportion becoming dry will be much more; most will be dry within the next year.

MEDICAL TERMINOLOGY

Enuresis — is the term used to describe lack of bladder control in a person who has reached an age at which control is to be expected. *Nocturnal enuresis* means night-time wetting ie. bed wetting (which is the subject of this book). *Diurnal enuresis* means day-time wetting. It is much less common than bed wetting. A small amount of dribbling and dampening of the pants is common in young school children but it does not cause such problems as night wetting and generally clears up speedily.

Intermittent enuresis — is the commonest sort of wetting in which the child has, or has had, occasional dry nights.

Secondary (or acquired) enuresis refers to a child who has been reliably dry for a year or more and then starts to wet again. It is sometimes also called 'onset' enuresis.

HOW THE BLADDER WORKS

Urine is made in the kidneys and passes down the two tubes, ureters, to the bladder where it is stored until being passed along the outgoing pipe, the urethra. The urethra is short in girls and longer in boys as it includes the length of the penis.

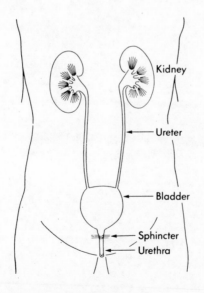

Kidney

Ureter

Bladder

Sphincter
Urethra

Fig. 1 Diagram of the urinary tract

If we drink only a little we pass very little urine, because our bodies use up some water all the time. If we drink much it is likely to be more than our bodies need and we get rid of it in the urine. Other waste products of the body are excreted dissolved in the urine, and therefore it is healthy to drink plenty so that the kidneys have an easier job in getting rid of the body's waste products.

In babies the bladder is small. It grows as the body grows and can hold more as the child gets older. The nerves controlling the bladder come from the bottom of the spinal cord but are influenced by messages from the brain. In infants the nervous connections are not well established but by the age of 5 the nervous system is mature, in full working order, and messages from the brain are able to influence control of the bladder. They can make the muscular walls of the bladder contract, and the sphincter muscle relax so that the urine is forced out along the urethra and the bladder empties.

THE DEVELOPMENT OF DRYNESS

Newborn babies pass urine frequently. They void (empty their bladder) whether they are awake or asleep but they are dry in between ie. their bladders are capable of holding a certain amount of urine and they do not dribble between each act of voiding. By the age of one month some babies begin to wake up, and some to give a cry, before or during voiding. The intervals between voiding and the length of the dry period become longer.

At the age of 15 months the child is likely to point to wet pants and puddles. Soon afterwards he may awaken at night after wetting and cry to be changed. He probably has a word which he uses to describe urine (and it is the same as that whcih he uses to describe faeces).

Between the ages of 1½ and 2 years most children are telling their mothers when they have wet themselves. They learn to tell the difference between urine and faeces and have a different word for them. At the age of 2 they may shout out when voiding and, a little later, *before* voiding. At that moment they are recognising the sensation of a full bladder. By the age of 2½ most children make known their need to pass urine. Girls tend to develop the skill earlier than boys.

The next stage is for the child to be able to delay voiding; even though he recognises the sensation of bladder fullness he can hold on for a short while, before having to void. At this age, providing that he can walk and has no restrictions from nappies or clothing, he is able to get to an appropriate place and pass urine. He can then be dry by day.

Three-year-old children are often proud of going to the lavatory on their own and they tell everyone about it. Some tend to hold on a bit too long and have accidents particularly when they are busy at play. By the age of 4 children are connoisseurs of lavatories and report in detail on the different features of a new lavatory. By the age of 5 the interest wanes and soon afterwards the child is insisting on shutting the door tight for complete privacy before voiding. It is at about the age of 5 that most children are able to start voiding even when their bladder is not full so that parents who want their children to pass urine before going out can encurge their child to do so. By the age of 5 the complex coordination between the nerves and the muscles controlling the bladder has developed and reliable dryness is possible.

Dryness by day nearly always comes before dryness at night. A few months after a child has become reliably dry by day he is likely to be able to be dry at night. Most children acquire the skill of dryness at night between the ages of 3 and 3½ but, as with all skills, there is a wide range of normal variation. Just as a few children may walk as early as 8 months of age and some normal children as late as 24 months of age so there is a wide range of normal variation in the development of dryness. It is important to remember that if the *average* age of becoming dry at night is 3¼ years then it means that half of all children will be dry before that age and that half will become dry *after* that age. Those that become dry after that age are not abnormal they are just later than average (in the same way half of us are taller than average and half of us are shorter than average, but not abnormal). By the age of 3½ years, 75 per cent of children are dry at night most of the time, many of these have an occasional accident when especially tired or ill.

Though some children suddenly achieve dryness and remain dry, many become dry gradually, the number of wet nights gradually diminishing over a period of months.

How do children become dry?

Children become dry by day gradually but we do not really understand how they manage to become dry for a 12-hour night, many not even needing to awaken to pass urine. It seems to be a natural animal skill: lions do not urinate in their dens, nor birds in their nests, even pigs have a special lavatory corner of the sty which is separate from their sleeping area.

Dryness at night does not depend upon special training it is a natural habit that emerges spontaneously — at different ages in different children.

Prevention of bed wetting

Since dryness at night develops spontaneously, the parents' job is to ensure that any 'training' or 'potting' regime they use for their convenience does not interfere with the normal emergence of dryness. Most regimes are harmless; only those that involve too much enforcement, punishment or stress are likely to interefere with the child becoming dry naturally. It is particularly important that pressure to become dry is not put on the child too early, before tha bladder is mature and the mechanism ready. If either parent wet the bed after the age of 5 it is more likely that the child will be ready to be dry at night later than usual (see p. 9). Furthermore, if the child is generally slow at acquiring all skills (e.g. walking and talking) he is likely to be ready for dryness later than usual.

When and how to try without nappies at night

The child usually provides the clue, by commenting on wet beds (or nappies) and by wanting to be dry. For some this will be about the age of 2½ for others 3½ or older. It is unlikely that he will be dry by night if he is not dry by day. Often the child will have shown that he can be dry while asleep by going dry during a short day-time sleep.

The time is then ripe for explaining to the child that you know he can be dry. Get him to urinate before getting into bed, discard night-time nappies and use pants or pyjama trousers, and tell him he can be dry. If he is dry in the morning give him a kiss and show him you are pleased (not by extravagant reward, but by simple pleasure — after all you told him you expected him to be dry). Tell him he will be able to go on wearing pants instead of nappies at night now because he has grown up. Occasional accidents will occur but the interval between wet nights will increase steadily.

If he is wet, accept it in an unworried way saying 'Never mind — I think wou will stop wetting soon, we'll try again tonight'. If the child is wet every night for 3 weeks (or any period that causes laundry problems or other difficulties) do not be too disappointed or show it. He is not ready to be dry, but will be soon; tell him he will be better off with nappies for a few months but that when he tries again in 3 months' time he will find it easier to be dry because he will be older. Avoid blame, avoid scolding, avoid punishment.

Remember that boys, first-born children, children whose parents wet the bed, and children who are slow learners, tend to be ready to be dry later. Postpone trying to get them out of nappies at night as long as you can (without too much inconvenience) and until the child seems ready to be without nappies. But do not wait too long — always have a go before 4 years of age.

Do not try without nappies if the child is ill, in a strange place or about to go on holiday or to hospital. Choose a time when he is well and life is the usual hum-drum routine. (And if your family and home are one of the many which stagger from crisis to crisis, then choose one of the least tempestuous times).

WHAT CAUSES BED WETTING?

The mechanism for becoming dry develops at different ages in different people. Part of the variation is because of our inheritance, the way we tend to take after our parents. Nearly three-quarters of school children who wet the bed have one or both parent who themselves wet the bed after the age of 5. Boys and first-born children wet the bed more often than girls or second and subsequent children.

Apart from the family tendency there are a number of factors which tend to produce bed wetting, and an even larger number that parents suggest as a possible cause.

Is it deep sleep?

Although some bed-wetting children do seem to sleep very deeply, research has not shown that most bed wetters sleep particularly deeply. And certainly many very deep sleepers either awaken to get up and pass urine, or alternatively can hold on until they awake in the morning. Most children who sleep deeply do not wet the bed.

Bed wetting is not the result of dreaming a lot. Most people dream for up to a fifth of their time asleep. Bed wetting hardly ever occurs during that dream time, though many of us can remember an odd occasion when it did.

Is it because of nervous or emotional disturbance?

Most children who wet become upset and at times depressed by the wetting. Often the wetting causes family unhappiness and rows, but these are more often the result of the wetting than the cause. However, once such stress and unhappiness is present in the child or family the wetting is more difficult to get rid of.

It is true that children with rare severe psychiatric illness commonly wet the bed, but most children who wet do not have such mental illness.

Is it because of naughtiness and laziness?

No. Wetting is unpleasant and degrading, children want to get rid of it and to have self respect. Some may adopt a 'don't care' attitude at home to their families, but you have only to see how seldom their friends know about the bed wetting to realise that the child is ashamed of it and wants to be dry.

Is it because of disease of the bladder or kidneys?

If a child is usually dry by day, and can pass a normal stream of urine it is highly unlikely that bed wetting is the result of any disease. Moreover if the child has had the occasional dry night during the previous year you can be sure that the mechanism to achieve dryness is healthy and ready. If the child is ill, feverish, dribbles urine all the time (day and night) or has pain you should consult your doctor.

Is it because of faulty toilet training or other harmful influences in early life?

Children, like most other animals, become dry spontaneously without training. In a few cases it seems that over-enthusiastic 'toilet training' at too young an age may predispose to wetting later on. Another link with later wetting is that of serious stressful events in early life. A serious stress, such as break-up of the parents' marriage or home, or prolonged stay in hospital, or separation from the mother, if it occurs during the period when night dryness would usually be acquired (ie. 2½—4 years), interferes with the development of dryness; so does the arrival of a new baby in the family. Subsequent bed wetting becomes more likely.

Is it because he is unintelligent?

Most children who wet have normal intelligence, though children who are seriously slow at learning any skill whether it be talking, writing or reading do tend to be slow at acquiring dryness also.

If the child learns most skills at the usual age, he is not unintelligent regardless of whether he still wets the bed. A boarding school headmaster when asked if he allowed boys who wet the bed to enter the school replied: 'Certainly, they provide most of my scholarship winners — and anyway they soon stop'.

Is it because of a small bladder?

Children who wet hold less urine in their bladders than those who are dry. Their bladders are not structurally small, they *can* hold more, but the child has the habit of not holding on for long when the bladder is half full. A small bladder is not in itself a reason for wetting. Many people who have structurally small bladders and have to pass urine very frequently can still be reliably dry in between, and do not wet the bed.

Is it because of the parents' attitude?

Wetting can persist if the parents attitude and approach is inappropriate. A sympathetic yet confident and encouraging approach is best (p. 17).

11

The following are nearly always unhelpful:

— Too much anger, scolding or punishment.

— Promise of lavish reward for dryness. It creates too much tension and though we acquire new skills well under a little stress, a lot of stress interferes with new skills developing.

— Repeatedly referring to the child as 'the one who wets the bed'. Children tend to fulfil their parents expectations; they perform best if they hear their parents saying they do something well not badly. Therefore, even in private, constant referral to a child as a bed wetter is unhelpful and such labelling in public is disastrously cruel.

— Removing the incentive to be dry. The normal simple incentive for the child to stop bed wetting is the wish to be grown up and rid of an unpleasant habit. Many caring and conscientious mothers mistakenly provide an opposite incentive to stay wet. When the child wets the bed they go to the bedroom, change him and cuddle him and, quite often, let him spend the rest of the night cuddled up in the parents bed. Such a child has very little incentive to be dry — for it will mean an end to cosy nights in mother's bed.

Most children who wet the bed do so because that is the way they are made. Very often they are taking after their parents. Their bladder and the nerves to it mature later than those who are dry early. For those who are later than average the worry of still wetting and the upset it sometimes causes in the family seem to make it even more difficult for the child to become dry. For a few children, severe stress in the pre-school years has made the acquisition of dryness difficult and, if acquired, not very secure. For an even smaller number severe behaviour disturbance or illness is the cause.

Perhaps those of us who become exasperated by a child's bed wetting and complain 'Why does he do it' should reflect for a moment that it is after all remarkable that people can unconsciously control their bladder while asleep. I do not know how we do it, yet *in the end children do stop wetting the bed*.

DISEASES
THAT CAUSE
BED WETTING

Most children who wet are healthy people who have no disease. Normal young children who are usually dry may have a wet bed when suffering from tonsillitis or any other illness, but the wetting stops when they are well again.

Bed wetting is occasionally a sign of disease. The two main groups of disorders are:

1. *Urinary tract infection.* The bacteria in the urine cause inflammation of the bladder and urethra. The irritation may make the person void very frequently and wet at night or during the day. The infection is detected by a laboratory test of the urine, and can be cured easily.
2. *Increase in volume of urine.* In some rare disorders of the kidneys or of the endocrine glands, the kidneys cannot concentrate the urine and so they produce an excess of dilute urine. The sheer volume of this imposes a strain on the bladder for it has to cope with more than it is accustomed to, and wetting may result. The chief examples of these disorders, diabetes and severe kidney disease, are rare in childhood and are usually accompanied by many other features of general illness.

An additional group of children who wet are those unfortunate ones who are born with a defect of the spine or of the nerves to the bladder or a defect of the bladder itself.

They will have wet all the time, day and night, and will not have had any period of dryness. They should receive specialist help early.

The child who wets is usually a healthy child attending school normally and leading a full life. It is unlikely that any disease is responsible for that child's wetting. The features that should make you consult your doctor earlier for a check on your child and his urine include:

— Wetting during the day as well as at night.
— If he is unwell with fever, pains, loss of appetite or other symptoms.
— If he can not pass a normal stream of urine and dribbles urine much of the time.
— If wetting starts in someone who has previously been reliably dry for over a year, over the age of 5. Dryness that is acquired very early in life often does not last, but the child who is reliably dry over the age of 5 develops bed wetting much less often and should be assessed by your doctor.

'Strong' urine

Urine is described as 'strong' if it is either dark yellow, very smelly or cloudy.

The commonest reason for dark urine is that it is concentrated. If we do not drink much, and particularly if we have perspired a lot because of hot weather, a feverish illness or exercise, the kidneys save water for the body and produce concentrated strong urine. A less common reason for dark urine is when the kidneys are excreting the colouring in things we have eaten, in confectionary, vegetables or medicines. Dark urine does not irritate the bladder and does not cause wetting.

Dilute pale urine which we produce when drinking plenty has almost no smell when fresh. Concentrated urine has only a mild smell when fresh. However, when it is left in the air or is soaked on to clothes or bedding it becomes stale and develops a foul smell. Unfortunately, children who wet are likely to wet their clothes or their bedding and the smell of the stale urine makes their parents think the urine is particularly strong.

If a bottle of fresh urine is held up to the light it looks clear. But as it stands and cools down the normal chemicals which are excreted in the urine may sediment out and make it cloudy or even produce a deposit at the bottom of the bottle. This is more likely with a concentrated sample of urine. It is normal.

An uncommon cause of discoloured, smelly, cloudy urine is an infection of the urinary tract (eg. cystitis). Such urine is cloudy and smelly as soon as it is passed — before it becomes stale. Urinary tract infection sometimes causes wetting.

HOW TO HELP THE CHILD WHO WETS THE BED

Since many children are not ready to be dry early, it is unwise to use any of the methods discussed in the next few sections before the age of 4. For young children the methods should follow the encouragement approach given on page 7. Bed wetting in a child aged 3¾ is a nuisance, but it is not a disorder. Be patient.

A great many different approaches and remedies have been tried over the centuries. Some of them help one child but not another; therefore, it is often a case of trying out different methods according to what seems suitable for your child and is least trouble for your home.

What attitude should the parents take?

This is very important. Parents should be confident, encouraging and patient. The child should know that the parents know, and expect, that he will become dry. They must steer the middle course between too much concern which makes everyone over-anxious, and a completely lackadaisical attitude which could make the child think that wetting was not a problem and not an inconvenience. Do not show disgust at sodden bed clothes or urine, but make sure he does not think you enjoy nights of changing wet bed clothes and days of washing them.

Many children are comforted by knowing that bed wetting is common and that other children share their problem. If there are 35 children in your seven year old's school class you can say with some certainty that 'at least two other children in your class wet the bed — they don't like it either so they don't talk about it, which is why you don't know who they are'.

Tell your child of someone (perhaps yourself or a relative) who wet when they were your child's age and who became dry.

What about punishments or rewards?

Most children who wet the bed want to be dry and do not require promise of reward. Extravagant promises such as 'We will all go on holiday to Majorca when you stop wetting' create too much tension, which interferes with the development of dryness. Similarly, punishments are likely to be inappropriate — the child cannot be deliberately wetting while asleep.

Lifting and awakening?

Many parents on their way to bed 'lift', or awaken, their child and persuade him to pass urine. If this prevents a wet bed later then it is worthwhile. It does not train the child to be dry, indeed most children barely wake up as their parents lift them on to a potty or the toilet.

Calendars, diaries and star charts

An interesting, colourful record card of dry nights can be a useful form of encouragement for a child, as well as a helpful record for the parent or doctor who is trying to work out how quickly the child is becoming dry. Children enjoy sticking a coloured star on a big calender or record card 'for a dry night'.

Alternatively the child can have a picture cut-out or transfer and be allowed to stick on another object each time he has a dry night. The emphasis is on the successful nights, the dry nights. Don't start putting a cross (or a skull and crossbones) by the wet nights.

Should drinks be restricted?

No. It does not usually make any difference, and normal drinking is a healthy and enjoyable habit. It is true that drinking a vast amount of fluid may cause wetting. The child who has 3 bottles of coke last thing at night is more likely to have a wet bed (and bad teeth) just as is the man who has 10 pints of beer. Normal drinking is all right.

Can the bladder be trained?

Some children who wet empty their bladders frequently during the day. They go to void many times in a morning, sometimes several times in one hour. Such children are more often girls. The child with a bladder that it not used to a large volume of urine may be helped by *interval training* which accustoms the bladder to hold on to larger volumes and stretches the bladder. Interval training takes time and trouble. Set aside a week for it. Explain the plan to your child and on the first day go with her to the lavatory to get her to pass urine. Use an alarm clock or timer and every half hour until bed time see that she goes and voids. On the second day make her go to the lavatory every hour. Increase the interval by 30 minutes each day. If she wants to go in between times discourage her or distract her. Tolerate the occasional accident but carry on trying to keep to time. By day 5 she will be up to 2½ hours, if she can manage 3-hour intervals on the next day that is even better. See how long she can hold on. Quite often if the child can have a few days voiding every 2½ to 3 hours she will at that stage stop wetting the bed. The bladder has become used to holding more urine.

Should the child be made to change the bed and wash the sheets?

Perhaps you should first ask yourself 'do I ask him to be responsible for changing and washing his daytime clothes?' If your answer to that is 'no', then it is unwise to 'rub his nose in it' by forcing him to be responsible for washing his bed clothes. But if, as in most households, your child takes some role in normal chores, whether it be washing up or cleaning, then it is fair to involve him to a small extent in the chores that result from his bed wetting. He needs to know that it is a nuisance for everyone, but not be disgraced by it.

Do not deliberately exaggerate the trouble involved in bed changing and laundry — make use of plastic mattress covers* and washing machines. It would be cruel to force him to wash his sheets by hand as a punishment if you have a washing machine in regular use.

Are drugs, tablets and medicines good treatment?

No. Ancient writings, dating back to the years before Christ, and modern research show that although a vast number of different drugs have been used for bed wetting, most do not work. Some seem to work — because children who wet are spontaneously becoming dry all the time (one in seven per year see page 1). Others seem to work because of the important power of suggestion on the child and family. The feeling that something positive is being done encourages the family to be hopeful, the worries to be less, and the child to be dry. But most of the time a dummy tablet given with the same sales talk, would be as effective.

There is one group of drugs that have been proved to be more effective than dummy tablets. These are the tricyclic

---

*It is worth getting a really strong one. Some cheap ones tear easily and do not weather the nightly flood too well. Strong ones can be obtained for about £1.50 (in 1980) from many stores including Boots and Mothercare.

drugs; e.g. imipramine (also known as Tofranil) and amitryptiline (e.g. Tryptizol). These are powerful drugs which can only be obtained on a doctors prescription. Like most powerful drugs they sometimes have unpleasant side effects — affecting mood or sleep or causing a dry mouth. Although many children who are prescribed one of these drugs become dry within a few days, most of them start wetting again when the drug is stopped, so that the drug treatment is nowhere near as effective as it at first seems. Another reason why doctors are reluctant to prescribe tricyclic drugs is that they are particularly dangerous if accidentally taken in excess. They are one of the most important and serious causes of childhood poisoning in Britain. Many of us are careless in our homes with tablets and medicines, and when we keep them on the top shelf of an unlocked kitchen cupboard an inquisitive toddler can climb up, sample them and poison himself. Therefore, if a doctor prescribes these as tablets or medicine for your child do keep them locked up away from any young child in your family or from visiting children.

Since drug treatment for bed wetting is often ineffective and potentially dangerous do not try to persuade your doctor to prescribe drugs for your child, when much better treatment rests with the general methods described earlier, or with the buzzer alarm described in the next section.

What about other unconventional treatments?

A great many different treatments have been used to cure bed wetting. The treatments vary according to the country, the culture and prevailing medical (or witch doctor) practice, for instance today in China acupuncture is standard treatment for bed wetting. It is reported to cure a fair proportion of bed wetters, but not as many as we can cure with our methods. There are many people who have been cured by hypnotism, special diets, allergen avoidance and other unusual treatments. It is difficult to measure the true value of some of these treatments because nearly one in seven children become dry within the next year without any treatment, and a higher proportion become dry with help regardless of its form (the mere suggestion of help and the comfort and confidence aroused by it tend to achieve cure).

If you are considering embarking on unconventional treatment for your child, or yourself, do ensure that it is unlikely to:

1. Cause harm
2. Cost more money than you can afford
3. Impose restructions on life to such an extent that normal activities are hindered or happiness jeopardized.

Apart from that — Good Luck!

Sore bottoms and rashes

Children who wet inevitably spend some time lying in night clothes or bedding soaked in urine. Fresh urine does not hurt the skin, but stale urine does. Particularly if the child has a sensitive skin, the child may get sore skin, blistering and a rash of the buttocks and thighs. The ways of helping are similar to those of easing a baby's nappy rash:

— Washing the buttocks and thighs each morning, and drying carefully, are essential, and also will prevent the child being teased as 'smelly' at school.
— Changing the wet pyjamas and bedding as often as is practicable, because the dirty clothing irritates the skin. Wash and rinse them thoroughly.
— Creams rubbed on each night help to protect the skin and to soothe it. Many are barrier creams, which prevent urine coming into direct contract with the skin, combined with an antiseptic which helps to stop the urine becoming putrid and irritant; (e.g. Syl, Siopel and Drapolene). Most chemists stock several effective creams. Ask for one that is useful for nappy rash or for ammoniacal dermatitis. For

very severe rashes you may need to get a stronger anti-inflammatory cream prescribed by your doctor.

BUZZER
ALARMS

In the last 20 years buzzer alarms have become an important and effective treatment for children who wet. They are widely used, and there is general agreement that although they may be quite a lot of trouble to use, that trouble is well worthwhile, because *they work*.

I shall refer to them as buzzer alarms. They are sometimes called enuresis alarms and the form of treatment referred to as conditioning therapy.

How do they work?

The child sleeps on a detector mechanism such as fine wire mesh or foil mats which are connected by wires to an alarm buzzer (Fig. 2). The buzzer is powered by a small battery. When the child wets, urine seeps down and triggers off the alarm (by completing the electrical circuit). When the buzzer alarm sounds the child has to get up out of bed, turn off the alarm, and go to the toilet to empty his bladder. At first the child tends to awaken slowly, after the bladder is empty and the bed is sodden, but after a few days he begins to wake up fast as soon as the first few drops of urine have triggered off the alarm. The wet patches become smaller, and then either he begins to awaken before the alarm has sounded ie. before he has wet, or alternatively he sleeps through the night without needing to wake up and void.

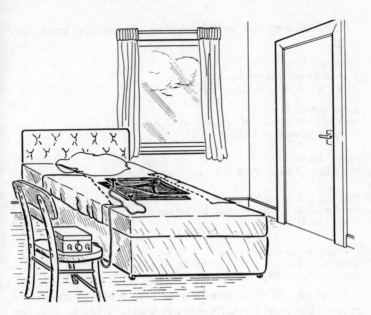

Fig. 2 Buzzer alarm set up in bed

Where can I obtain one?

It is most convenient to borrow one, because you are likely to need it for between 2 and 5 months. Some general practitioners have one or two to lend, many health centres and local authority school clinics have them and nearly all hospital paediatric (children's medicine) outpatient clinics have them. From these sources there is no charge: it is part of the National Health Service. There is the added advantage that usually there will be someone there to advise you about their use as well as to help with the general problems of bed wetting.

Some of the firms who sell buzzer alarms will hire them out. The hire charges are quite expensive (e.g. £8.00 a month in 1980) and considering how long you are likely to need the buzzer alarm it can be a better bargain to buy one. The least expensive reliable models cost between £15 − £20 (in 1980).

The following list includes buzzer alarms that are widely used:

Eastleigh Alarms
N H Eastwood and Son Ltd
70 Nursery Road, London N14 5QH

Astric Dry-Bed
Astric Products Ltd, 148 Lewes Road,
Brighton, Sussex BN2 3LG

Chiron Alarm
Down Bros., Church Path, Mitcham, Surrey

Headingley Enuresis Alarm
Headingley Scientific Services, 20 Cottage Road,
Leeds LS6 4DD

Wessex Transistorised Alarm
Wessex Medical Equipment Company, Alma Road,
Romsey, Hampshire.

Some of the firms produce several different models. A private buyer will usually manage well with the least expensive model. The expensive models tend to be more robust and to have extra fitments which are useful to a hospital department that is regularly lending them out to a succession of families each with slightly different needs. A silent awakener or vibrating alarm which is put beneath the child's pillow, is available for deaf children. It can be obtained from Headingley Scientific Services.

If you do decide to buy an alarm kit it is worth sending a doctors certificate or letter of recommendation with your order. That allows the firm to sell it to you without Value Added Tax, and therefore the total cost is less.

Setting up the alarm

If you borrow one from a clinic you will be shown how to set it up and probably given an instruction leaflet.

Involve the child at once. Make sure he understands it, and get him to help with setting it up. At the very least ensure that he is the person who checks that it is switched on each night when he goes to bed. Try setting it up during the day and test it by pouring a little water, with salt added, on the bed to trigger off the buzzer. (Ordinary water seldom works because it does not conduct electricity in the same way as salt water or urine.)

The detector mats should be placed in the middle of the bed, where the first wetness is likely to occur. If it is a very saggy mattress or bed it may be worth putting a board underneath the mattress to prevent the detector mats crumpling or slipping.

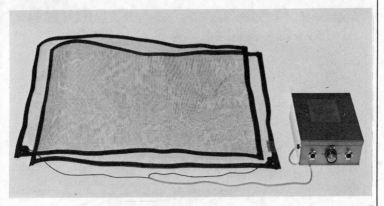

Fig. 3 Buzzer alarm kit which uses two mesh detector mats

Most sets of equipment use two detector mats (Fig. 3) which must not touch each other directly. They must be separated by a piece of material, part of an old flannelette sheet is suitable provided it has no holes in it and is big enough to cover the mats with plenty of overlap. Alternatively the mat can be put inside a pillow case to stop it touching the other mat directly. Some kits use a single mat, and are easier to set up (Fig. 4). The detector mats are covered with a sheet which is firmly tucked in round the whole mattress (Fig. 5). Then the bed is made in the usual way with the bottom sheet well tucked in to keep the detector mats in place.

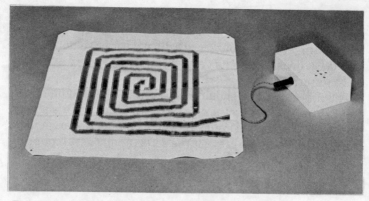

Fig. 4 Buzzer alarm kit which uses a single detector mat

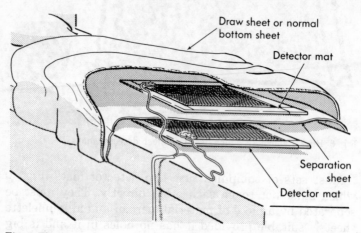

Fig. 5 The arrangement of mats and sheets when using a two-detector-mat kit

The wires from the alarm are clipped to opposite corners of the detector mats, one to the top mat and one to the bottom mat. The alarm is then put on the floor or on a chair out of arms reach from the bed, because the child must be made to get up out of bed to turn it off.

Use and care of buzzer alarms

The makers provide useful instruction leaflets, and include maintenance advice about replacement of batteries and how to clean the detector mats. It is important to follow these instructions carefully.

Are they safe?

Yes. The thought of electrical currents and alarms involving your child in bed may sound dangerous and raise fears of electric shocks, but they are not dangerous. The alarms are made under strict safety regulations. They are not, and must not be, connected to the electricity mains supply. They are powered by a small battery like that for a portable radio, and in fact can be considered safer than a small radio.

How old must the child be to use one?

Most children over 7 use the alarms sensibly and without much fear or trouble. They need parental help at the start. Adolescents and adults usually can manage on their own. Children under 5 tend to be frightened of it and it is better to wait until the child is older rather than create a lot of unnecessary turmoil and fear by trying to use it for a pre-school child.

Between the ages of 5 and 7 many children can use the alarm successfully provided they have sympathetic help. It depends on their maturity and ability to understand and co-operate with the treatment. If the child is generally a bit slow at learning or is emotionally immature it is best to delay using the alarm until he is behaving more like a 7-year-old. Most children over the age of 7 can use them successfully.

Does the child need his own bedroom?

It is best, if arrangements can be made, for the child to have a room to himself while using the buzzer so as not to awaken anyone else. It is not essential. The other occupants of the room may complain at first about the alarms, but they get used to it. The child with the buzzer should not share a bed during the course of treatment.

Each night as the child goes to bed he checks that the alarm is switched on. He has been told that he has got to 'beat the buzzer' and that if it goes off he must waken up as fast as possible, get up, switch it off and go to the toilet. The child should wear only a pyjama jacket or short nightie and must be nude from the waist down because one wants the first drop of urine to soak down and trigger off the alarm. Normal drinking is allowed.

Must the buzzer be reset after wetting?

Ideally, Yes. After the child has got up and been to the toilet the wet detector mats should be disconnected and replaced by dry ones and a dry sheet before the child returns to bed. The alarm should be reset so that another wetting incident will trigger it off. That is the ideal and it is worthwhile if you can manage it, but it is a hard task in the middle of the night. Since most children only wet once a night it does not matter too much if the mechanism is not reset in that way. Cure may take a little longer, but it will happen all the same.

Record keeping

A careful record is important and also encouraging to the child and family. If a record card has not been provided with the alarm you should make one. Here is an example (Table 1).

Encourage the child to fill in the card each morning. Parents will need to help young children but all children are capable of filling in part of the card. It is a good habit when filling in the card to check that you have remembered to turn off the alarm during the day.

Table 1 A record of buzzer alarm treatment. (This was the first week of use, and the child was reliably dry 6 weeks later.)

NAME: *David Higgins*

DATE OF STARTING TREATMENT: *September 10th*

Date	Dry (D) or Wet (W)	Time of alarm (ie. when wet)	Did the Alarm wake the child	Size of wet patch
10th	W	2.30	No	Bed soaked
11	W	1.10	Yes	2 foot
12	D	–	–	–
13	W	12.45	Yes	1 foot
14	W	?	No	Bed soaked
15	W	3.15	Yes	9 inches
16	W	12.30	Yes	1 foot
17	D	–	–	–
18	W	12.15	Yes	6 inches

For how long must the alarm be used?

It is best to continue using the alarm until the child has had 6 weeks (ie. 42 nights) without a single wet bed. For most children that means using the alarm for about 4 months. At the end of that time 4 out of every 5 children will be dry. It is common for the child to wet every night at first, but then dry nights become more common and the size of the wet patches on those wet nights becomes smaller. After starting to use the buzzer children usually have between 15 and 20 wet nights (and buzzes) before becoming dry. Some children become dry sooner, others later and they have to put up with more buzzes before dryness is reliable.

The first week of use

Buzzer alarms are excellent and effective treatment; therefore make sure you use them well. In particular, be prepared to take a lot of trouble and to put up with some inconvenience in the early weeks, especially the first week. Start using the alarm only when you can see a fairly settled 3 or 4 months ahead. Do not start if you are going to be moving house or going on holiday in 2 weeks' time. Do not start if you have illness or some other temporary time-consuming family crisis on your hands. Be prepared for an inconvenient 4 months. If you usually go away in your caravan most weekends in the summer then either stay at home, or delay starting treatment until you are at home for a few consecutive months.

It is in the first week or two that the child may need a lot of help. Be prepared for that. Listen for the buzzer yourself: providing he eventually awakens, gets up and turns it off, that is fine; but if he does not the parent must get up and rouse the child until he hears the buzzer and gets out of bed

N.B., the parent does not switch off the buzzer, but rouses the child to hear the buzzer so that the child is sufficiently awake to turn it off.

Should other treatments be combined with the buzzer?

The general attitude and approach to helping the bed wetting child are described on page 17. They are an essential part also of any special treatment. Since the alarm works as a result of wet beds it is usually best to stop 'lifting'. If, despite lifting, your child was still wetting the bed then you can continue to lift (as well as use the alarm) until he has almost stopped wetting. At that time stop lifting him, you may get an increased number of wet beds temporarily but improvement will soon occur. If your doctor has prescribed drugs for the bed wetting discuss with him the need to continue the drugs. It is likely that they can be stopped.

COMMON PROBLEMS AND DIFFICULTIES WITH BUZZER ALARMS

Not awakening to the alarm

This is common at first, and usually both child and parent claim it is because of deep sleep. It is worth remembering that if the alarm was sounding to wake him up to go off on holiday to the Costa Brava he would almost certainly hear it. It is difficult to wake up in the middle of the night and it needs practice and determination, but it is possible. At first a parent should go through and rouse the child as outlined on page 32, but the parent should make it clear that this is only a short term manoeuvre and that by, say, day 10 the child must be waking up himself. Therefore in the first week a parent may have to change bedrooms and sleep within earshot of the buzzer.

There are extension buzzers, extra loud buzzers and vibrating alarms available from special clinics, but in general the need is for more determination and co-operation rather than for extra loud alarms.

Failure of the alarm to sound

Check that the alarm is switched on, and the connecting cables plugged in. Check that the alarm works (p. 27). If it does not it may merely need a new battery. Otherwise return it to the clinic for repair (or if you have bought it, return it to the makers). If the alarm works when you test it but not during the night ensure that it is not because the child is awakening fast, switching off the alarm and going back to sleep. Talk to him and explain why he must not do that. Put the alarm further away from him so that he has to get right out of bed to turn it off. Look for disconnections or breaks. Check that the wire connectors are intact and that they are firmly clipped to the detector mats and the detector mats are intact. On some of the kits that use a single detector mat the coil of foil or wire strip may be cracked. It is common for a child to need an additional set of detector mats during a 4 month course of treatment.

Check that the detector mats are lying over the area of the bed which gets wet first.

False alarms

It is annoying for everyone when the buzzer sounds and the child has not wet. Possible causes are:

1. Detector mats touching each other. They should be separated and completely covered, with some overlap, by strong material such as flannelette. Mesh mats may become frayed at the edges so that fine wire prickles through the dividing sheet and forms a short circuit. Sometimes the offending section can be bound with tape; or a new set of detector mats may be needed.

2. Crumpled detector mats. Smooth them flat and bind the mats to the mattress tucking the covering sheet well beneath the mattress.

3. The connecting cables touching each other. It is helpful to connect the clips to different corners of the mats so that the clips don't lie directly above each other with the possibility of touching each other and establishing the electrical circuit which triggers off the alarm.

4. Perspiration. A pool of sweat can create electrical contact between the detector mats. Try using a thicker bottom sheet (ie. the sheet which covers the detector mats), or

thicker or double material between the detector mats. It may be that the bedroom is too hot and fewer bed clothes or an open window is the most appropriate solution.

Failure to void after awakening

The child who wakes up, switches off the alarm and goes back to sleep without going to the toilet has to be talked to and told that it will not work unless he does get up. The buzzer can be put as far out of reach as possible, if necessary using more cable to do so, on the basis that if he has to walk across the room to turn it off he is more likely to become thoroughly awake and to use the toilet.

Terror and confusion

Wild confusion when the alarm sounds is most likely in young and immature children. They may be helped, and the confusion overcome, by the mother being available at once to help the child find the alarm and turn it off. It may be justified for the mother to sleep in the child's room for a week. But if, after a week or two, the child is still confused and frightened by the alarm, it is better to abandon treatment temporarily, and to try again in 6 months when the child will be older and more able to cope with it.

For some children a low-voltage night light left on all night may be helpful.

No cure after 4 months

80 per cent of children who use the buzzer become dry within 4 months. By that time it is usually clear what to do for the minority who are still wetting. If the record card shows that the child is improving, that the wet patches are becoming smaller, and the number of dry nights increasing, it is reasonable to persist for another month or two. But for most of those still wetting after 4 months improvement is no longer occurring. Then it is best to abandon treatment for the time being, without blame or too much despair. Simply, decide to

give it a rest and to try again in 6 or 9 months time when the child will be a bit older and the bladder more ready to be dry.

One of the principles of helping children to become dry is to have short periods of determined action and encouragement. If that treatment spell is unsuccessful then stop bothering about it for a while and try again later. That is a much better approach than many months or years of half-hearted treatment.

Recurrence of wetting after cure

Once a child has been reliably dry for 2 months he usually stays dry. A few children who have cured themselves of wetting with a buzzer alarm start wetting again some months later. If that happens borrow an alarm again. Such children respond fast to the alarm, they already know how to use it and usually dryness becomes re-established and secure within a few weeks.

Very occasionally a child may have a second recurrence of wetting. If he has had two previous courses of the alarm and each has produced only temporary cure try a third course with 'overlearning'. Start using the alarm in the usual way, but when he has had 6 consecutive dry nights get him to drink a pint of liquid last thing at night. That makes it more difficult for him to be dry, and it forces the bladder to accommodate more urine. Temporarily it may result in wet beds and buzzes. Ensure that the extra drinking is continued for 4 weeks. Carry on using the buzzer until he has been dry for 5 weeks. The dryness should now be permanent.

WHERE
TO GET
HELP

In the first place consult you own doctor. He may wish to examine your child and test a specimen of urine. He will be able to advise you about the best management.

For young pre-school children your health visitor may be helpful and she and others at the child health centre have a lot of experience of young children.

Help can also be obtained from many health centres, local authority and school clinics for children.

If specialist help is needed the child is likely to be referred to a hospital paediatric outpatient clinic. Such referral to a children's specialist has to be via your general practitioner.

In many areas there are special clinics for children and adolescents who wet. Some are run by paediatricians, some by local authority or school doctors and other by psychologists who are experts at behaviour therapy. It does not matter who runs the clinic; if it is a special clinic for bed wetters there are likely to be experts there who can help.

ADULTS
WHO WET
THE BED

Although many adults have an occasional wet bed, it is uncommon for adults to wet frequently, and it is important for an adult to go to his doctor first, because a general health check and urine test is essential for adults who wet. It is more likely that a doctor will consider an X-ray examination of the kidneys and bladder to be needed for an adult than for a child. Providing the health checks are normal the principles of treatment are the same for adults as for children (see p. 17). Buzzer alarms are particularly effective for adults because they are able to understand them better than children. Some adults have difficulty awakening to the alarm at first and a relative or friend may be needed to help awaken them in the first week of alarm treatment.

The 25-year-old who still wets should not think that their wetting is impossible to treat or cure just because it has gone on for 25 years. Often the reason is that they did not get the right help at the right moment in childhood. Nevertheless they can become dry now. (In the last 12 months I have seen one lady of 28 become reliably dry; she was engaged to a man who did not know she wet the bed! And a sturdy coal miner aged 22 has now become dry after using the buzzer alarm for 3 weeks).

If you are an adult who wets the bed, go for help, and get yourself cured. You may keep it a secret from your friends, but do not let it stop you planning to get married. Do discuss it with your fiancé(e), get help, and remember that it nearly always stops anyway when you start sharing a double bed.

It may seem to you that there is no point aiming at a particular career because of the training and periods of residence that are involved and which could be difficult if you wet the bed. But bed wetting can be cured so do not let it interfere with your plans for a career or your life. Make normal plans and in addition get help for your bed wetting. It will stop.

Author's note
In this book I have mainly used the word 'he' when describing the bed-wetting child. This is not because of lack of concern for 'she' wetters: all deserve sympathy and help. It is because we males do wet the bed more often — but we eventually stop. I did.

OVERSEAS DISTRIBUTORS OF BUZZER ALARMS

Downs Surgical Limited:

Canada:
Downs Surgical Canada Ltd., 261 Davenport Road, Toronto, Ontario M5R 1K3.

U.S.A.:
Downs Surgical Inc., 2500 Park Central Blvd., Decatur, Georgia 30035.

Australia:
Downs Surgical (Australia) PTY. Ltd., 575 George Street, Sydney 2000, N.S.W.

Ireland:
Surgical Distributors Ltd., Gibralter House, Herberton Road, Dubin 12.

N H Eastwood and Son Ltd.:

Europe:
R R Pyle
PO Box 14 177, s-Gravenhague, Holland.

U.S.A.:
Electronic Monitors Inc., PO Box 8280, Forthworth, Texas 76112.

GLOSSARY

Glossary of terms used in this book or which may be used by doctors discussing bed wetting.

Buzzer (enuresis) alarm
   An alarm mechanism to cure bed wetting.

Conditioning therapy
   Special treatment used to alter behaviour, in this case to cure bed wetting by the use of the buzzer alarm.

Colony count
   A count of bacteria in urine which is done in the laboratory to detect urine infection.

Cystitis
   Urine infection within the bladder.

Cystoscopy
   An examination done under anaesthetic by a surgeon who uses an instrument telescope to inspect the inside of the bladder and urethra.

Cystourethrogram
   An X-ray picture of the bladder and urethra.

Diurnal enuresis
   Day-time wetting.

Dysuria
   Difficult or painful passage of urine.

Endocrine glands
   Glands in the body that produce chemical secretions (hormones) which control the body's function — e.g. the pancreas which produces insulin.

Ammoniacal dermatitis
   Skin rash, usually involving the buttocks, caused by stale urine.

Enuresis
Wetting occurring at an age when dryness should be expected.

Faeces
The waste products of the body excreted by opening the bowels.

Frequency
Frequent acts of voiding (bladder emptying), regardless of the amount of urine.

Hereditary
The transmission of certain characteristics from parent to child. Sometimes called a 'genetic tendency'.

Intravenous urogram (I.V.U.) *or Intravenous pyelogram* (I.V.P.)
An X-ray examination of the kidneys, which involves an injection of dye into a vein of the arm followed by a series of X-ray pictures of the abdomen which show the kidneys excreting the dye.

Micturate
To pass urine.

Micturating cystogram (M.C.U.)
An X-ray examination of the bladder. A catheter tube into the bladder is introduced along the urethra; dye is poured through it and pictures taken of the bladder before and during emptying.

Nocturnal enuresis
Night-time, or bed, wetting.

Primary enuresis
A term used to describe someone who has *never* been dry. Most children have had an occasional dry night and, more accurately, are said to have intermittent enuresis.

Pad and bell
Another name for the buzzer alarm.

Polyuria
Passage of large volumes of urine.

Pyelitis
Urine infection within the kidneys.

Renal
Concerning the kidney.

Secondary enuresis
Enuresis occurring after a period of a year or more of reliable dryness. Also called 'acquired' or 'onset' enuresis.

Sphincter
The muscles controlling the outlet from the bladder.

Tricyclic drugs
A group of powerful drugs used chiefly for the treatment of depression, and which by chance were found to be of temporary help to bed wetters.

42

Ureter
   The tube connecting the kidney to the bladder.

Urethra
   The pipe from the bladder to the outside (see diagram on page 3).

Urinary tract
   The excretory system made up of kidneys, ureters, bladder and urethra.

Urinary tract infection
   An excess of bacteria in the urine within the urinary tract which may cause illness or other symptoms including wetting.

Void
   To pass urine and empty the bladder.